10 FOODS YOU SHOULD NOT EAT

Author Annie B. Kelly

Copyright © 2020 Annie B. Kelly. All Rights Reserved.

No part of this publication may be reproduced, distributed, or transmitted in any form or by any means, including photocopying, recording, or other electronic or mechanical methods, or by any information storage and retrieval system without the prior written permission of Smith Show Publishing, except in the case of very brief quotations embodied in critical reviews and certain other noncommercial uses permitted by copyright law.

10 Foods You Should Never Eat

10 foods you should never eat. Your health depends on what you eat. Let me say it again your health depends on what you eat. This is true and you have to truly know what you are eating. Your health is one of the most important assets that you have in your life too. We will let you know about 10 foods you should never eat because these types of foods are not good for you at all. We will give you the details that you need so you can avoid them as much as you can too.

How does the body use energy?

Your body needs energy to function and grow. Calories from food and drinks give you that energy. Think of food as energy to charge up your battery for the day. Throughout the day, you use energy from the battery to think and move, so you need to eat and drink to stay powered up. Balancing the energy you take in through food and beverages with the energy you use for growth, activity, and daily living is called "energy balance." Energy balance may help you stay a healthy weight.

How many calories does your body need?

Different people need different amounts of calories to be active or stay a healthy weight. The number of calories you need depends on whether you are male or female, your genes, how old you are, your height and weight, whether you are still growing, and how active you are, which may not be the same every day.

10 Foods You Should Never Eat

How should you manage or control your weight?

Some teens try to lose weight by eating very little; cutting out whole groups of foods like foods with carbohydrate, or "carbs; "skipping meals; or fasting. These approaches to losing weight could be unhealthy because they may leave out important nutrients your body needs. In fact, unhealthy dieting could get in the way of trying to manage your weight because it may lead to a cycle of eating very little and then overeating because you get too hungry. Unhealthy dieting could also affect your mood and how you grow.

Smoking, making yourself vomit, or using diet pills or laxatives to lose weight may also lead to health problems. If you make yourself vomit, or use diet pills or laxatives to control your weight, you could have signs of a serious eating disorder and should talk with your health care professional or another trusted adult right away. If you smoke, which increases your risk of heart disease, cancer, and other health problems.

One sugary drinks: you have to be wary of sugary drinks, they taste good and all that stuff but you have to be careful because they are not good for your health. If you drink too much of them

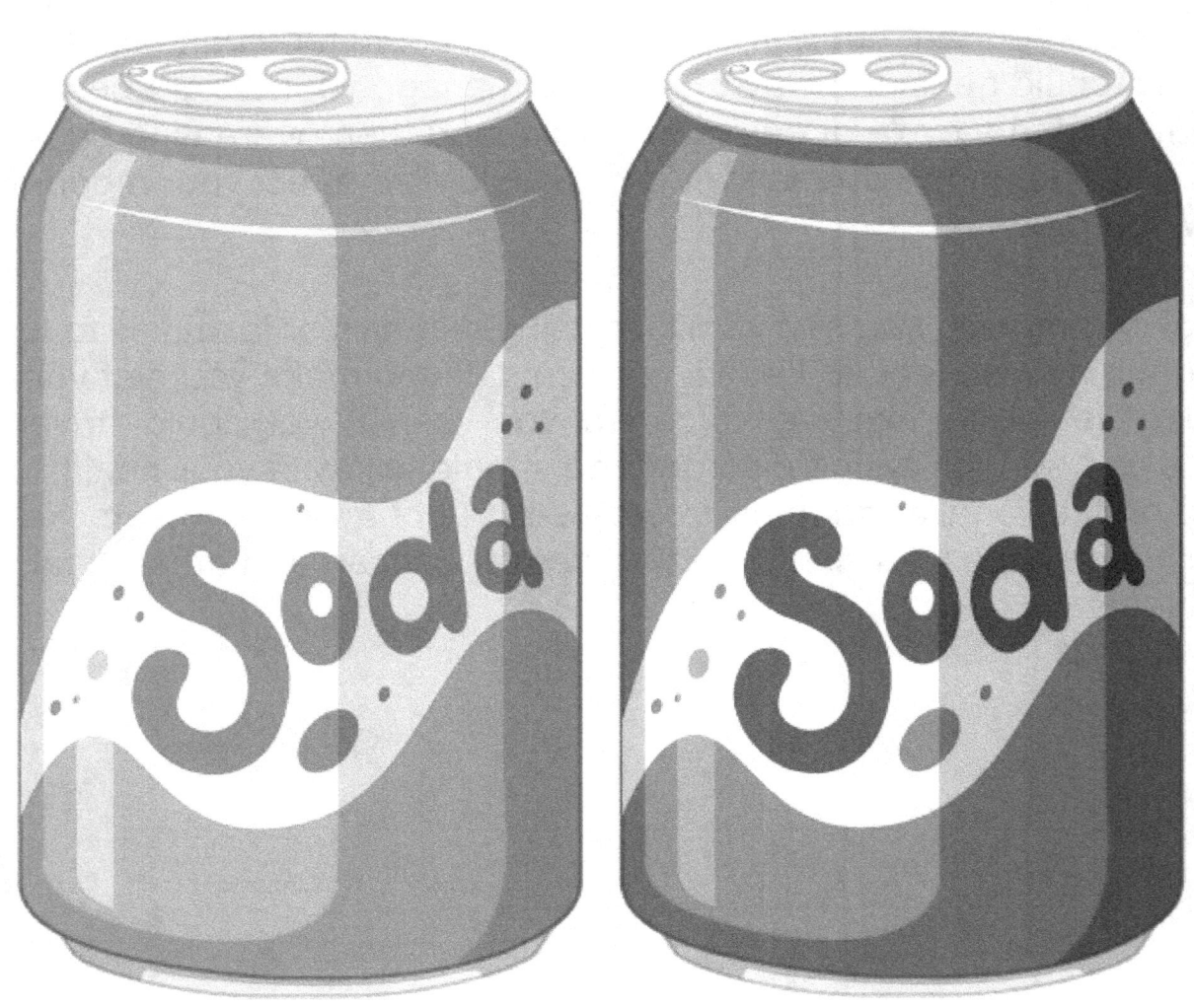

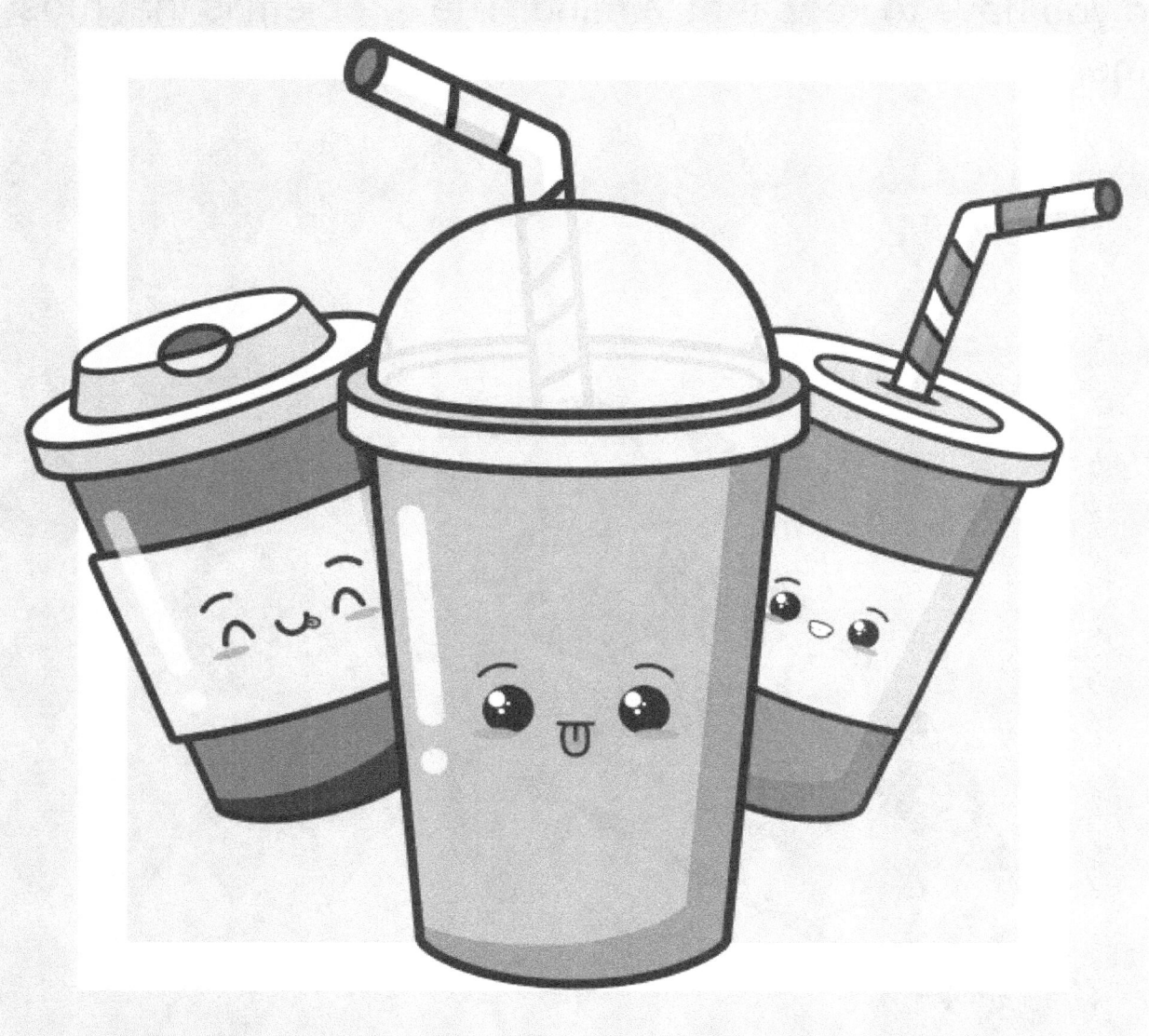

Two pizza: you have to be wary of pizza too. This is junk food and you have to keep that in mind. The problem is that most of them are made with unhealthy ingredients.

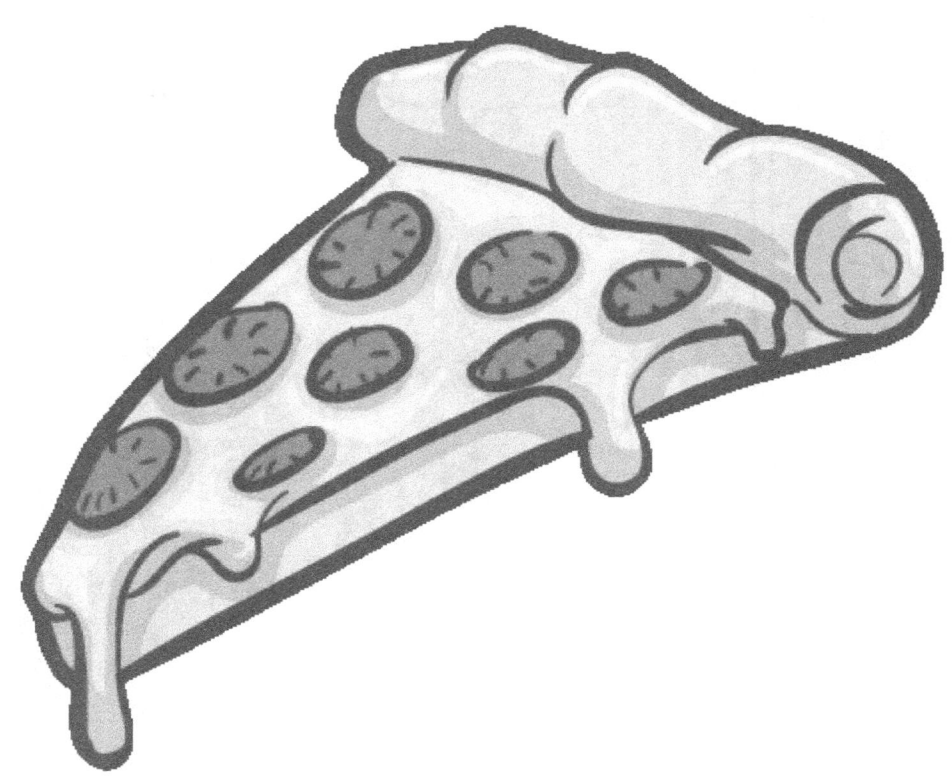

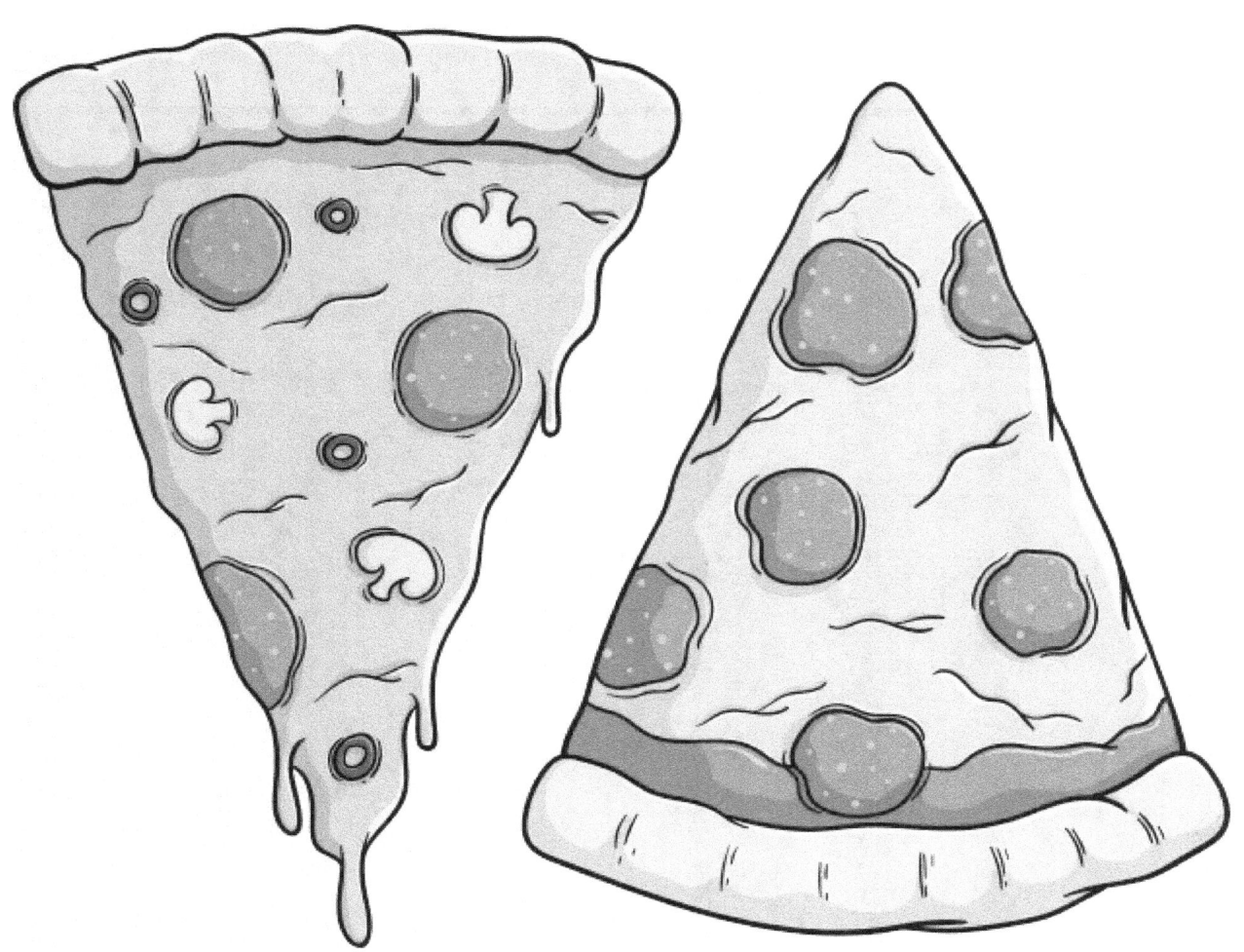

Four fruit juice: a fruit juice here and there from time to time it's not bad. But the problem is that these types of juices have tons of sugar most of the time.

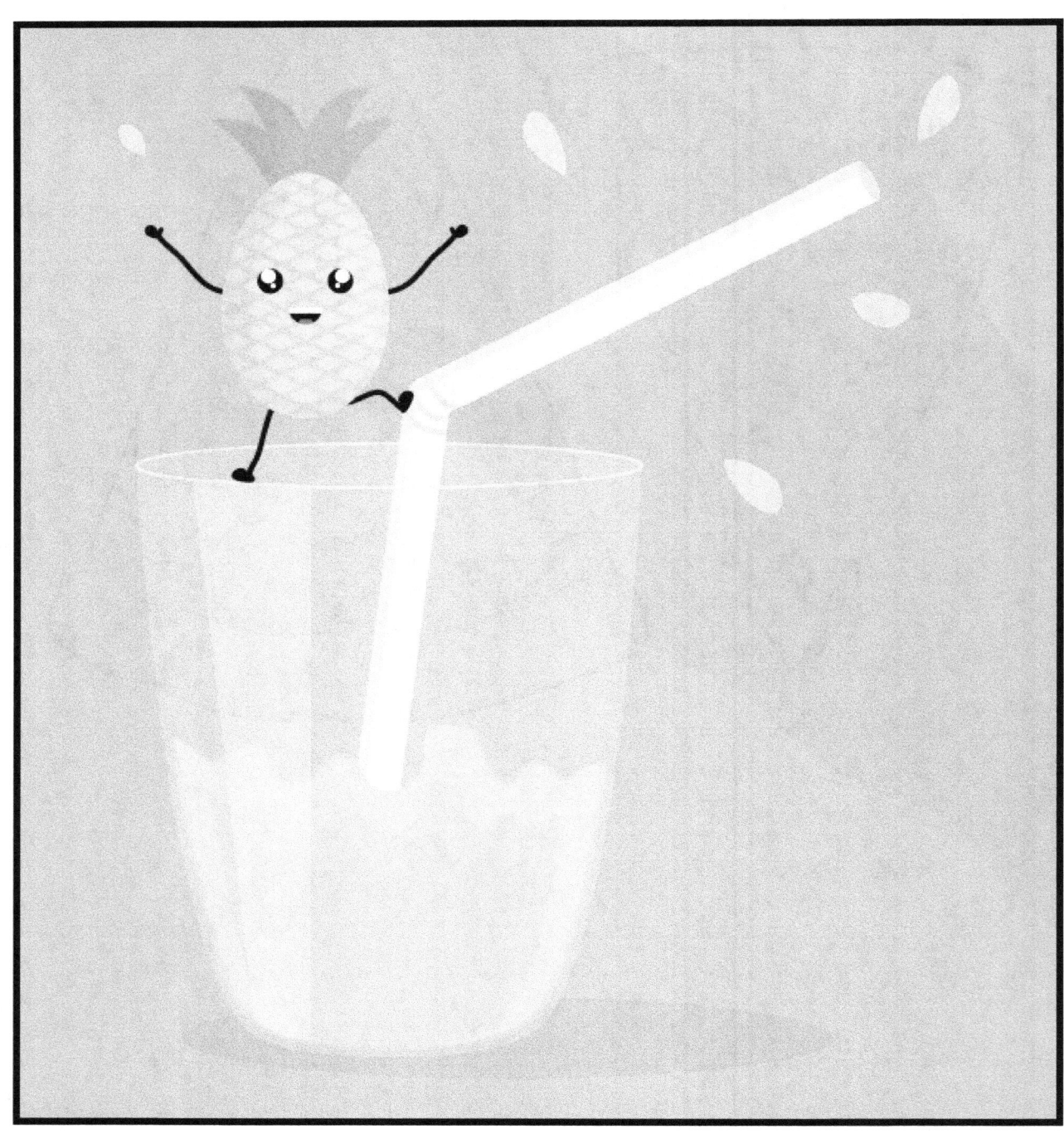

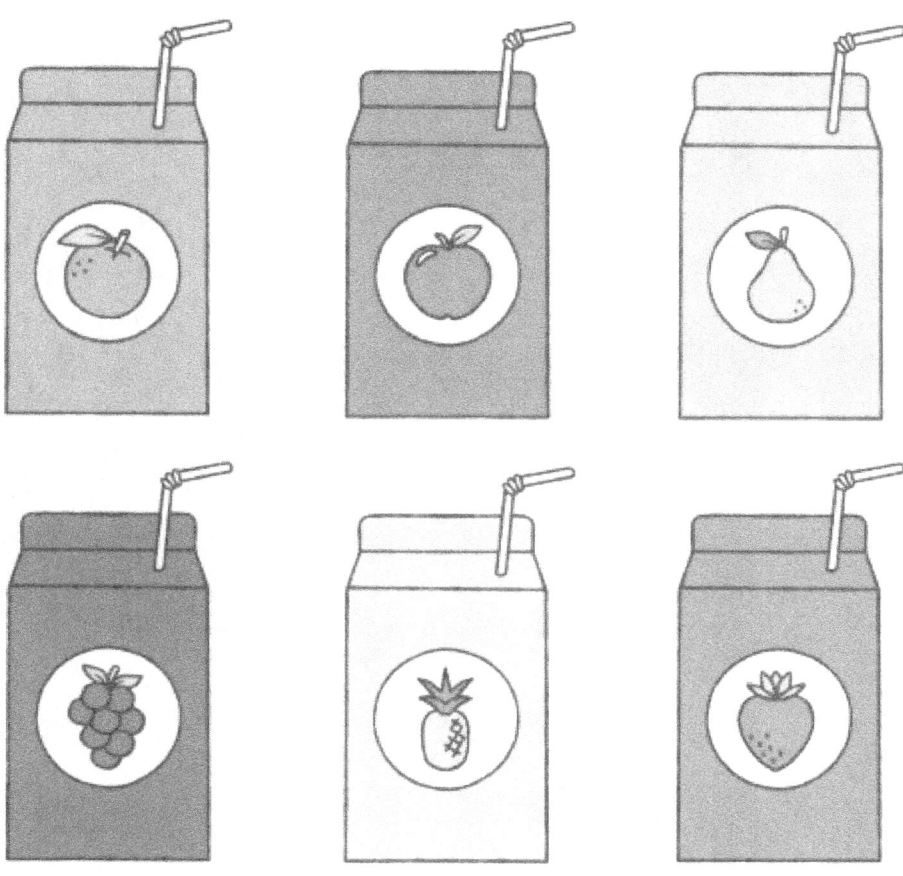

Three white bread: If you suffer from gluten sensitivity, white bread is not good for you at all. This bread is a starch and turns in to sugar.

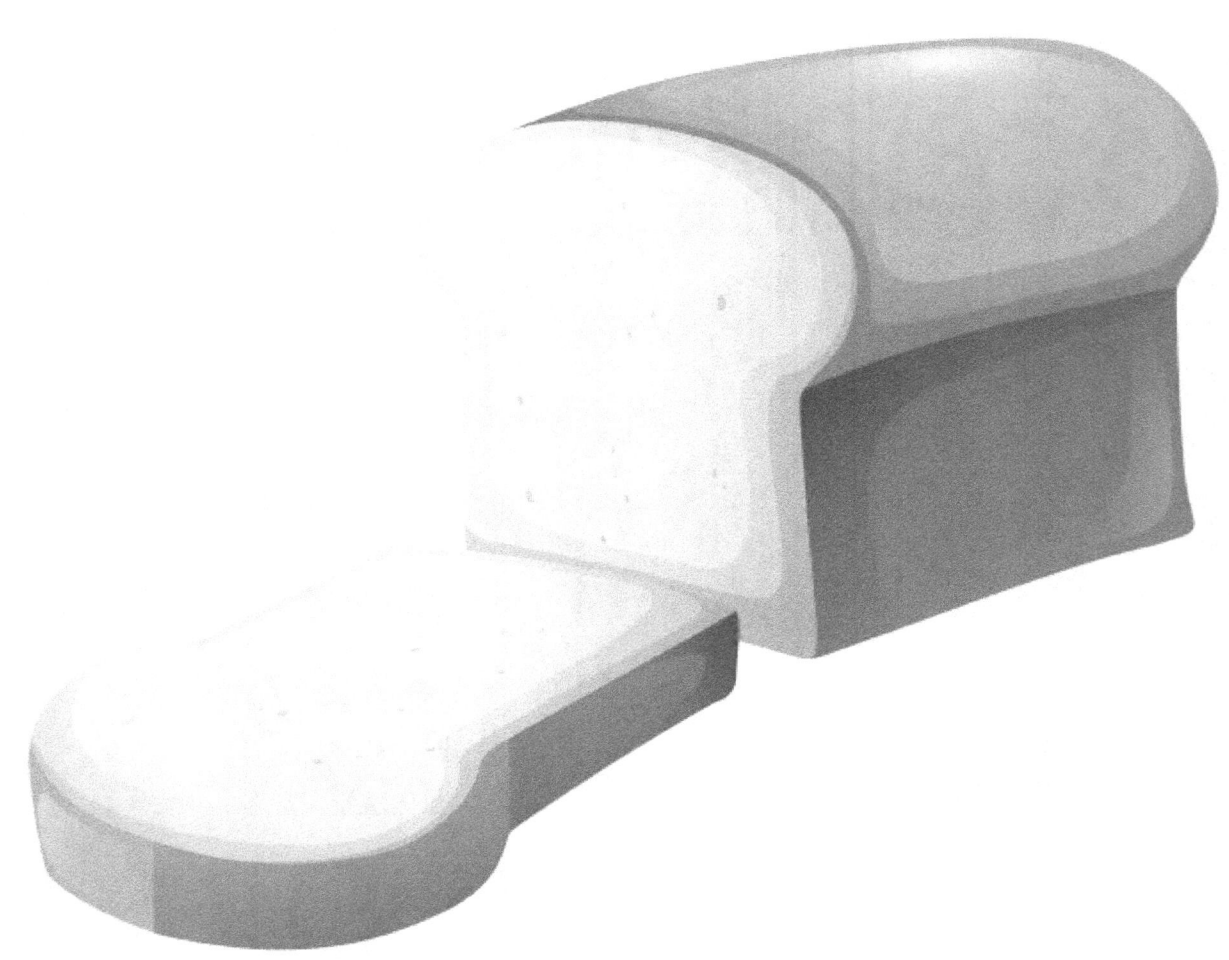

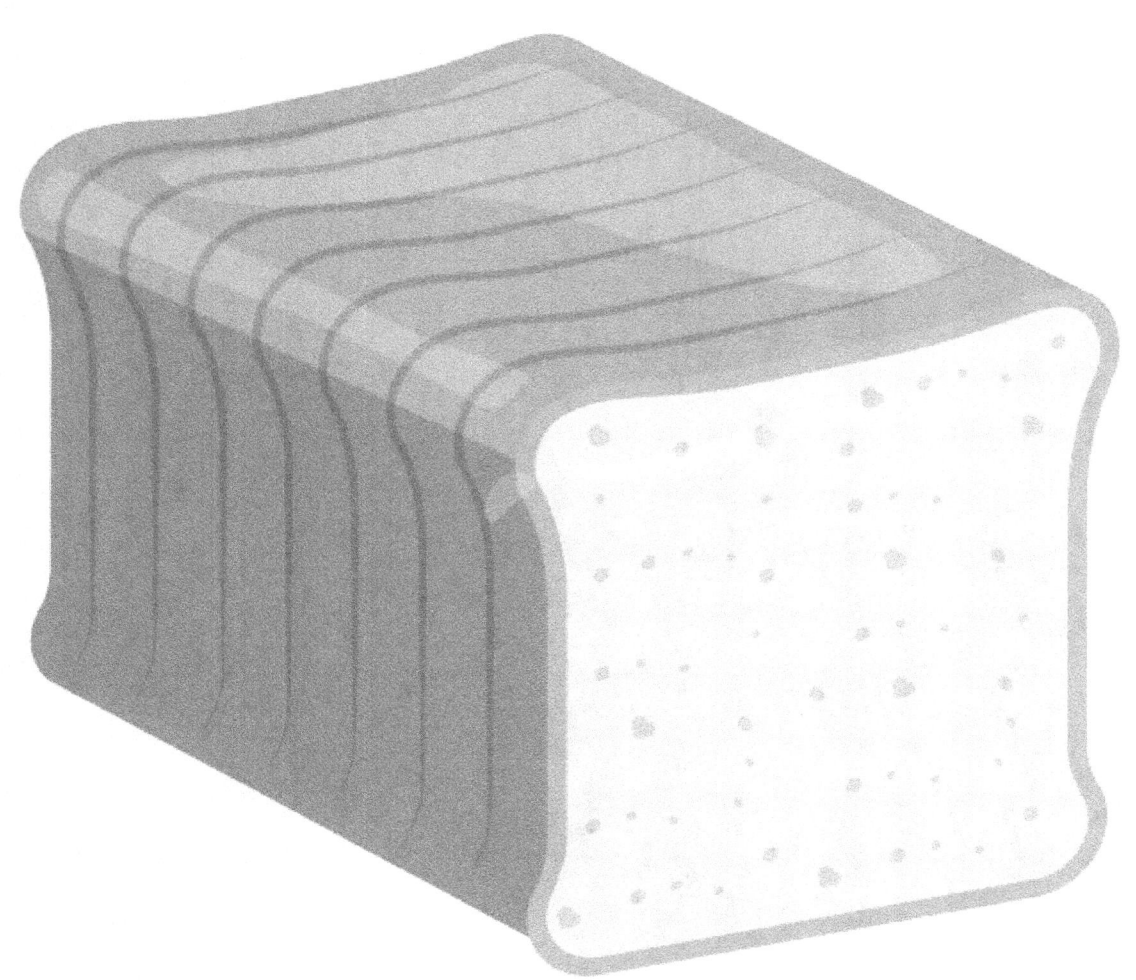

Five industrial vegetable oils: If you consume a lot of corn oil, canola oil or soybean oil, this might cause a problem to you when it comes to keeping your body healthy

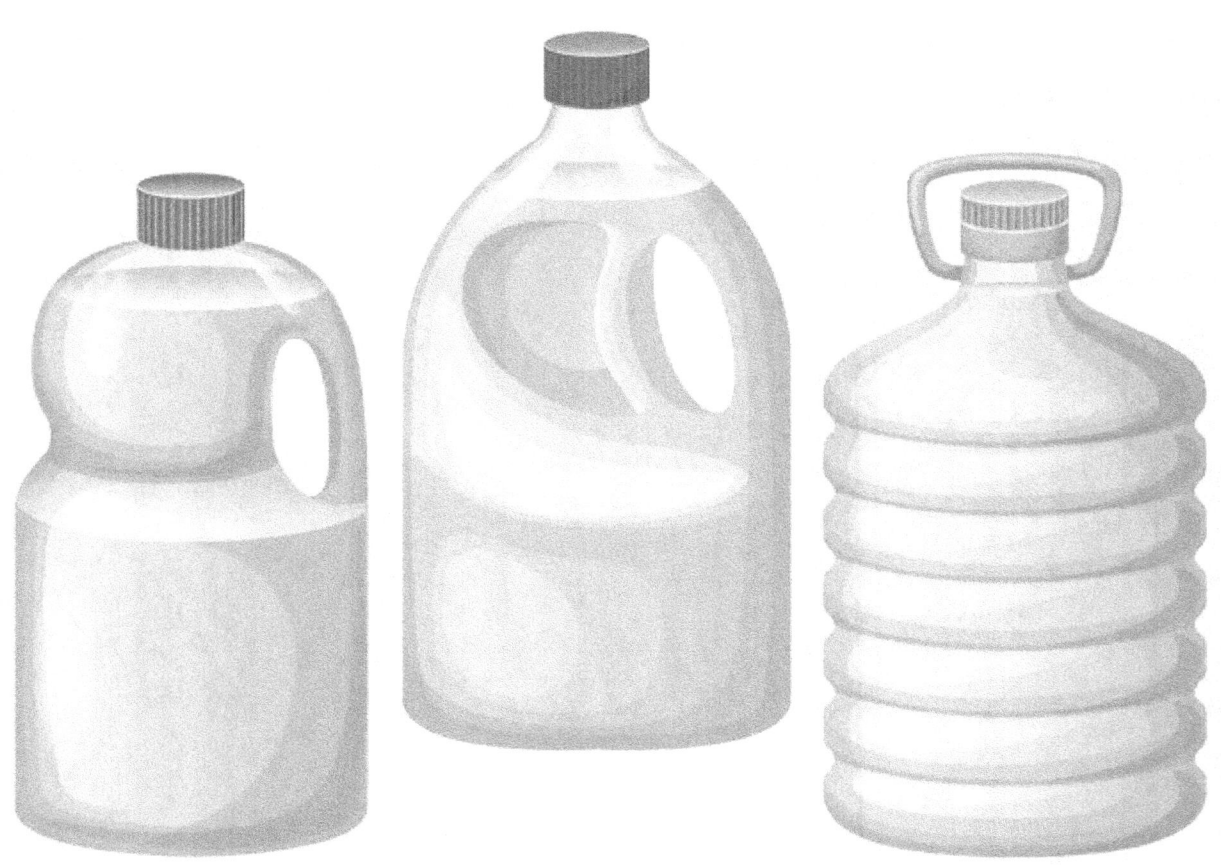

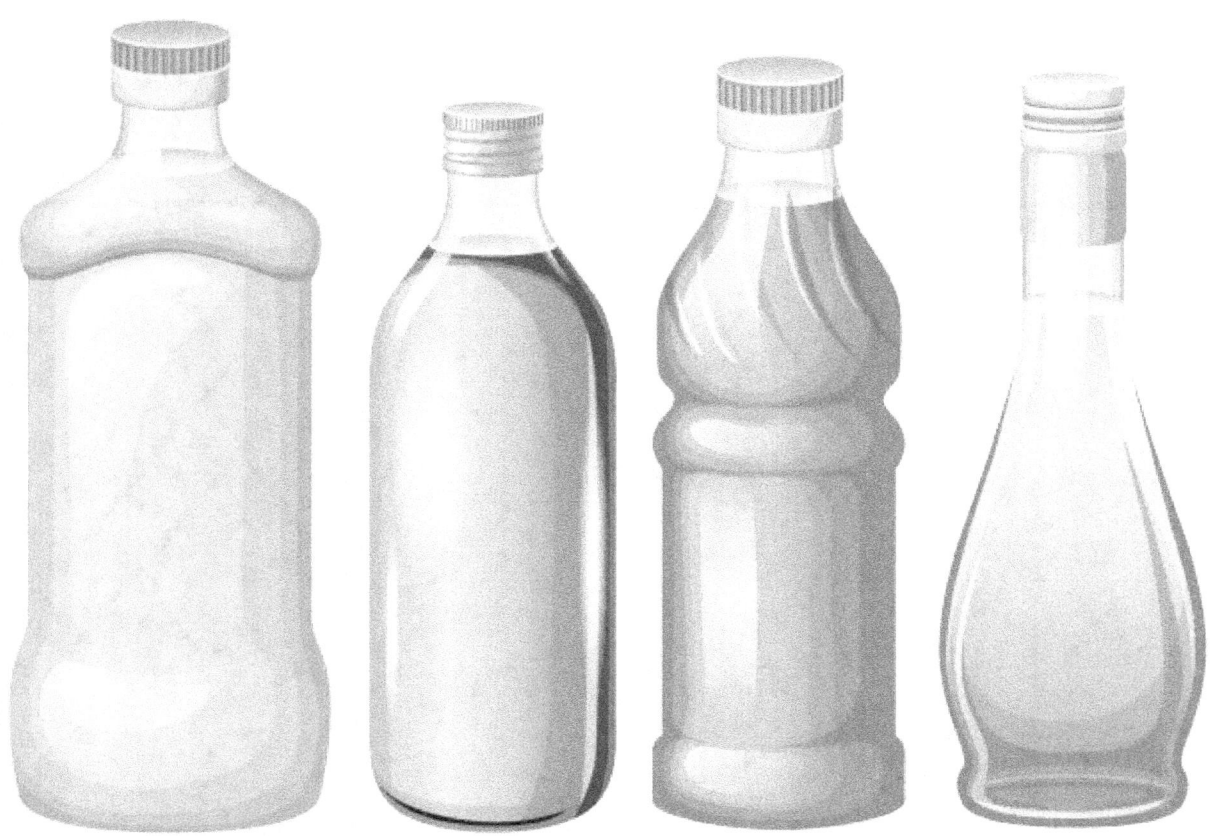

Six trans-fat: you need to avoid trans-fat as much as you can. The problem with trans fat is that it will raise your bad cholesterol which is not good for your health at all.

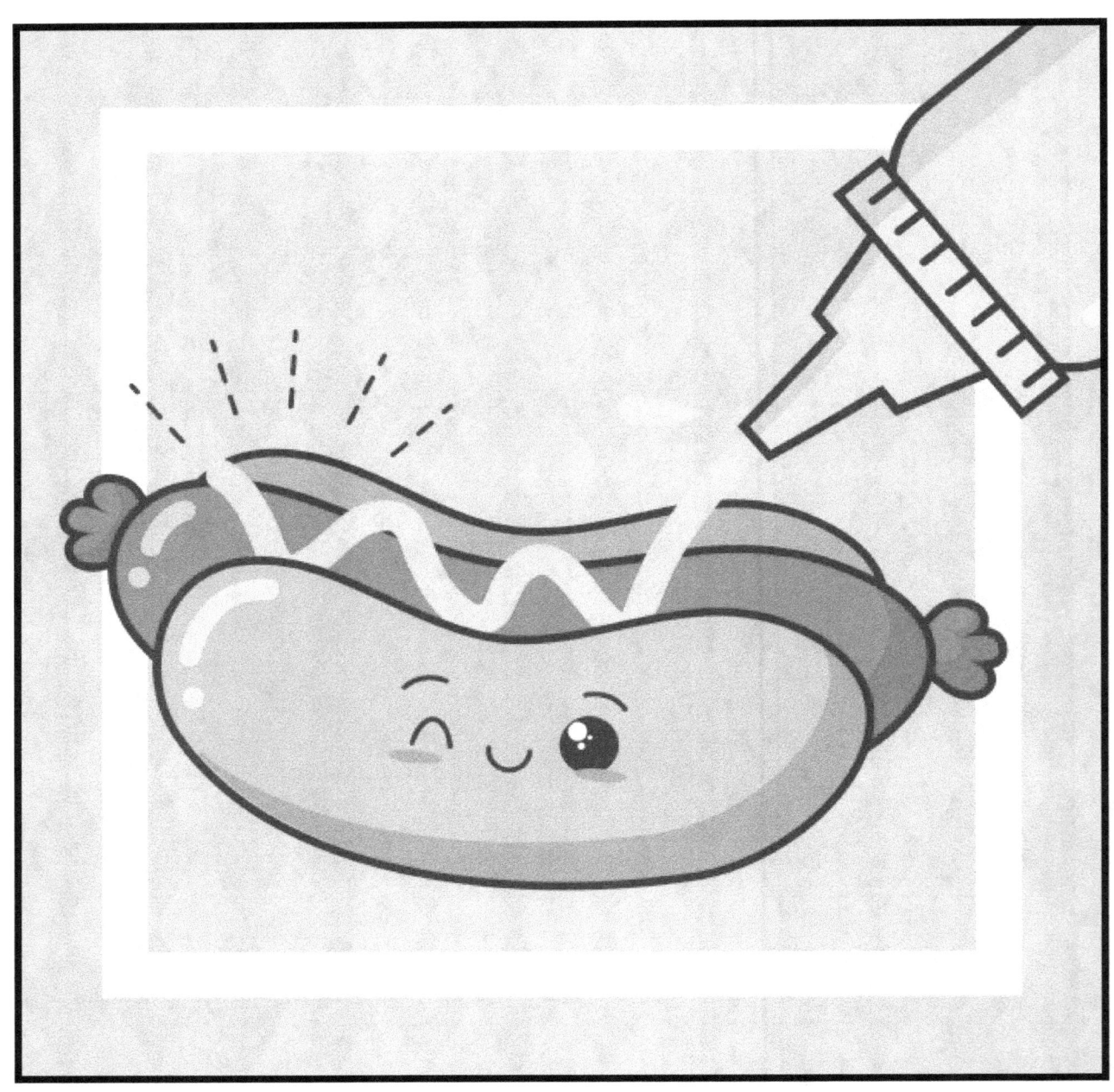

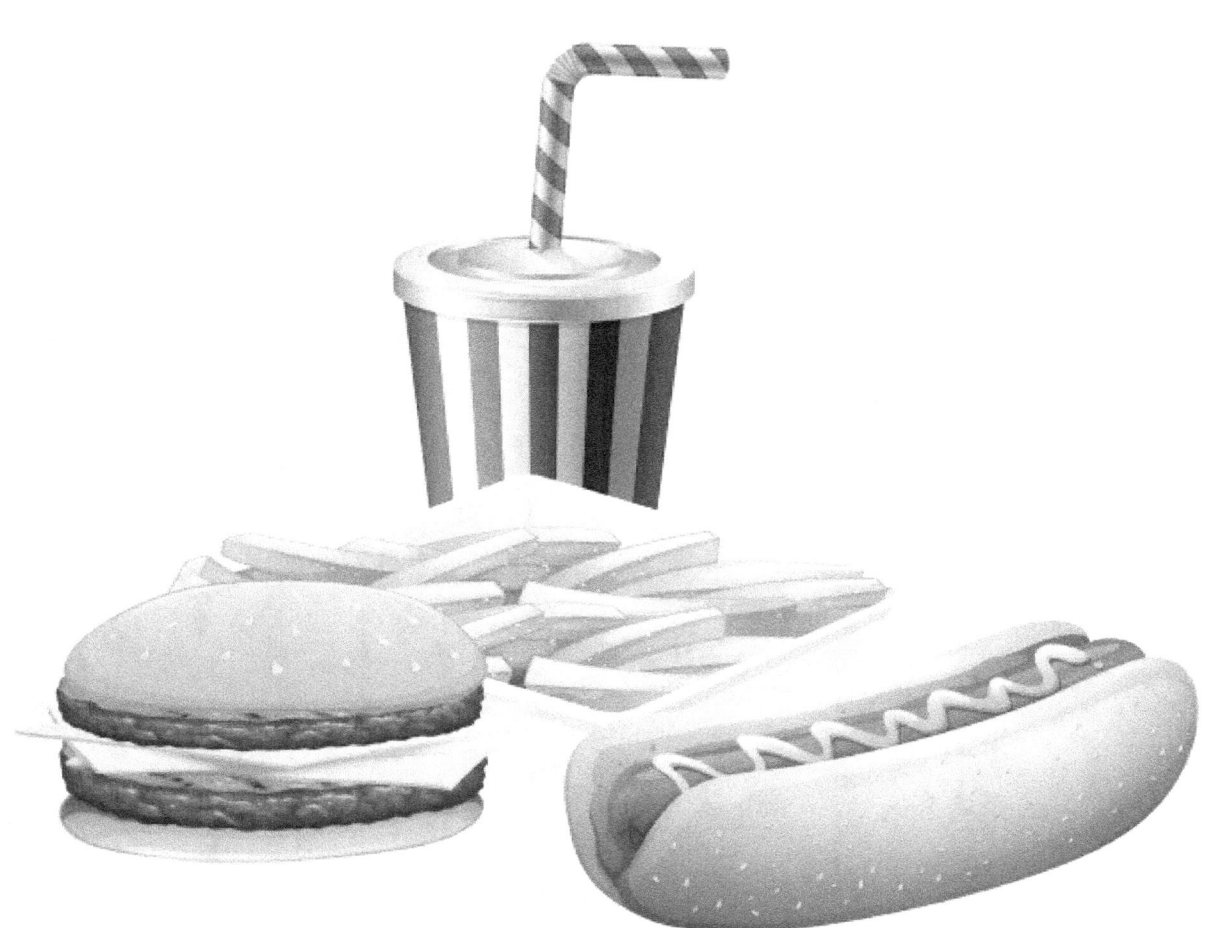

Seven Soylent protein: you have to avoid soy protein because this is not healthy food at all. The popular belief is that this food is good for you. But that is not the case.

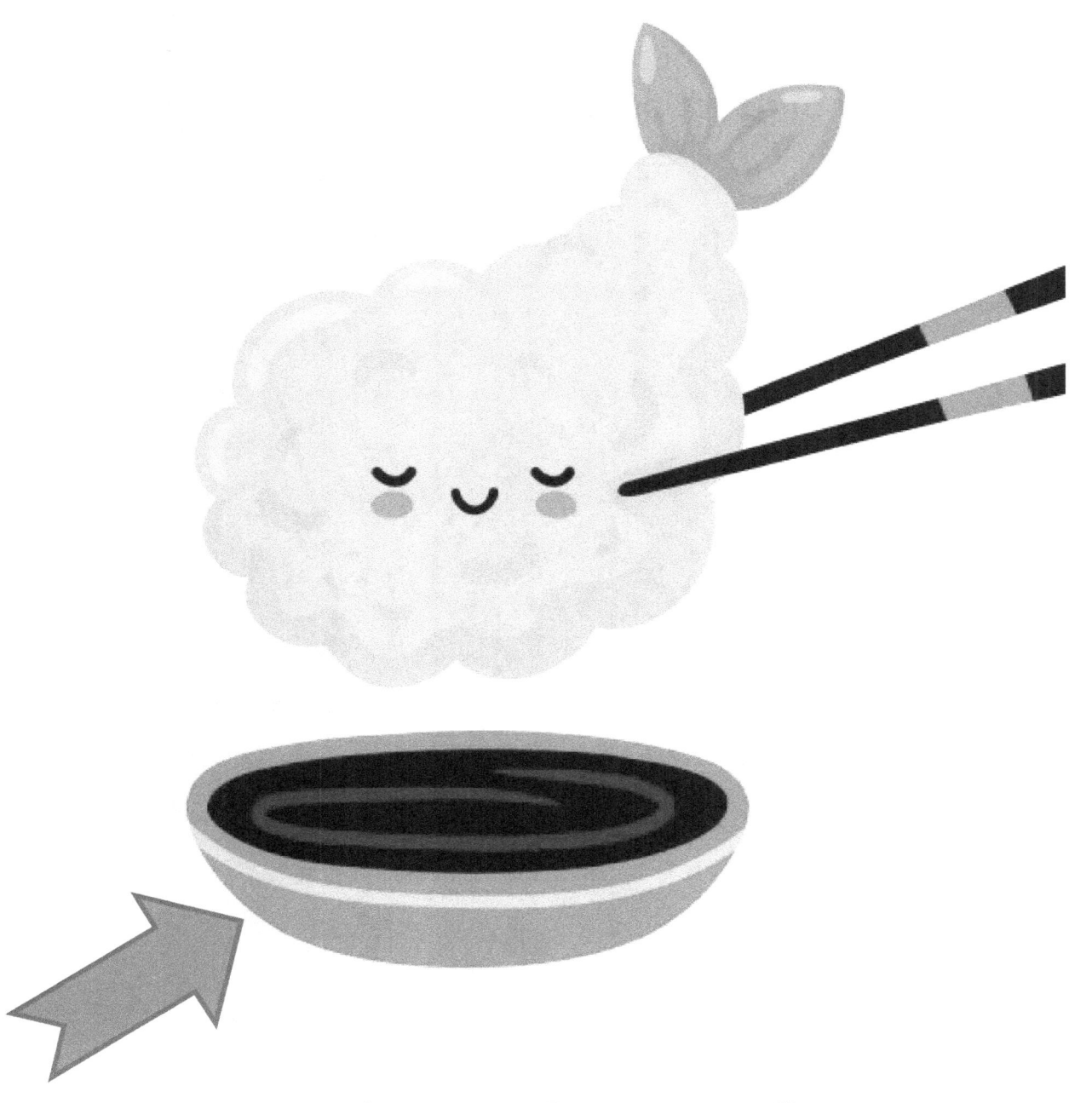

SOY SAUCE

Eight farmed fish: You have to understand that farmed fish is not good for you at all. Eating, tilapia and things like that it's not good for your health at all to.

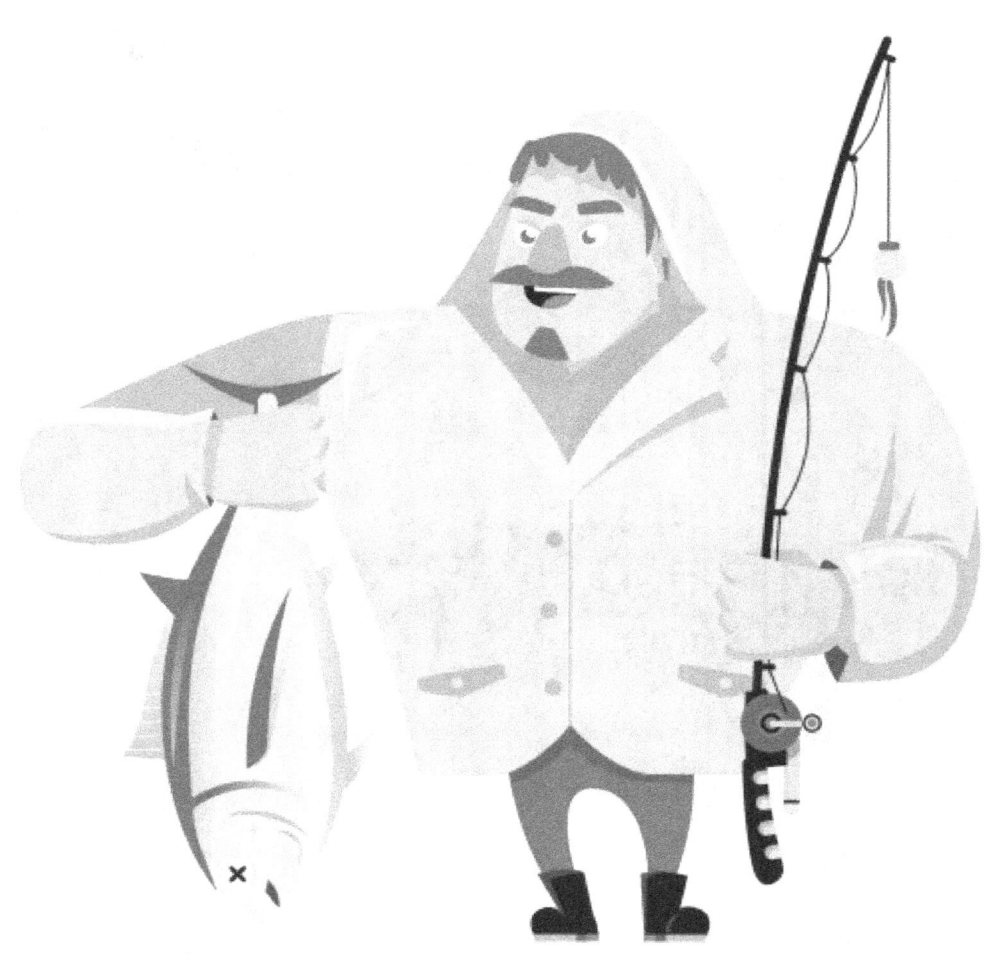

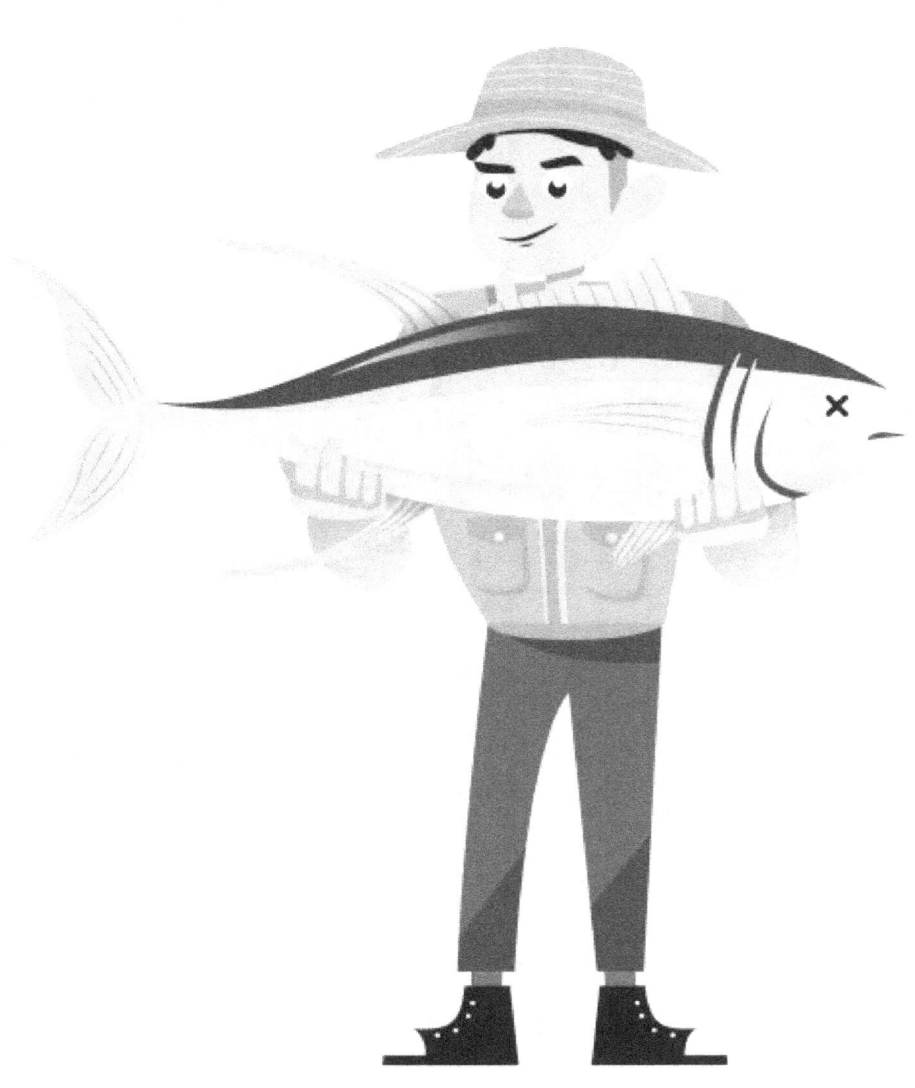

Nine, microwave popcorn: Do you love popcorn? If so, you are in a bad situation right away. You have to consume way less popcorn that you think because this food is not good for you at all if you consume too much of it. 10 factory farmed meat factory farmed meat is not good for you at all.

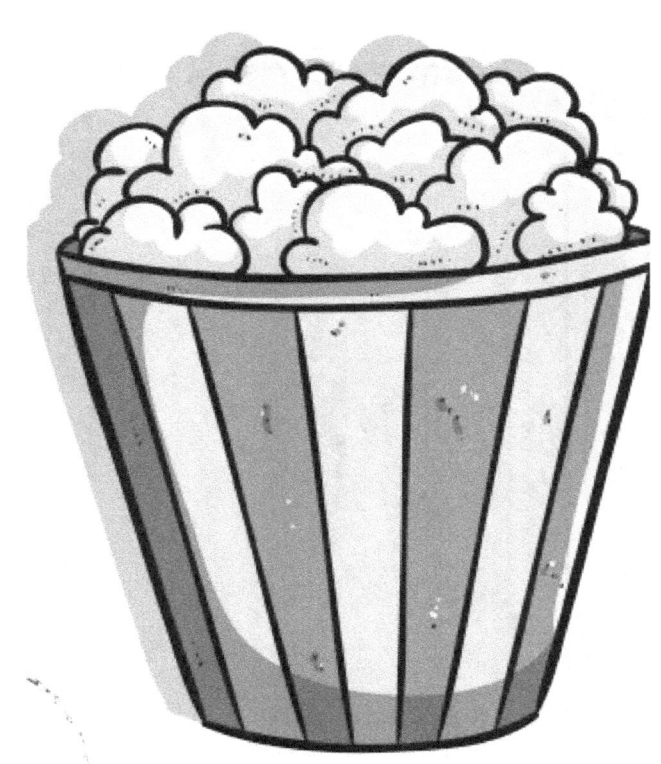

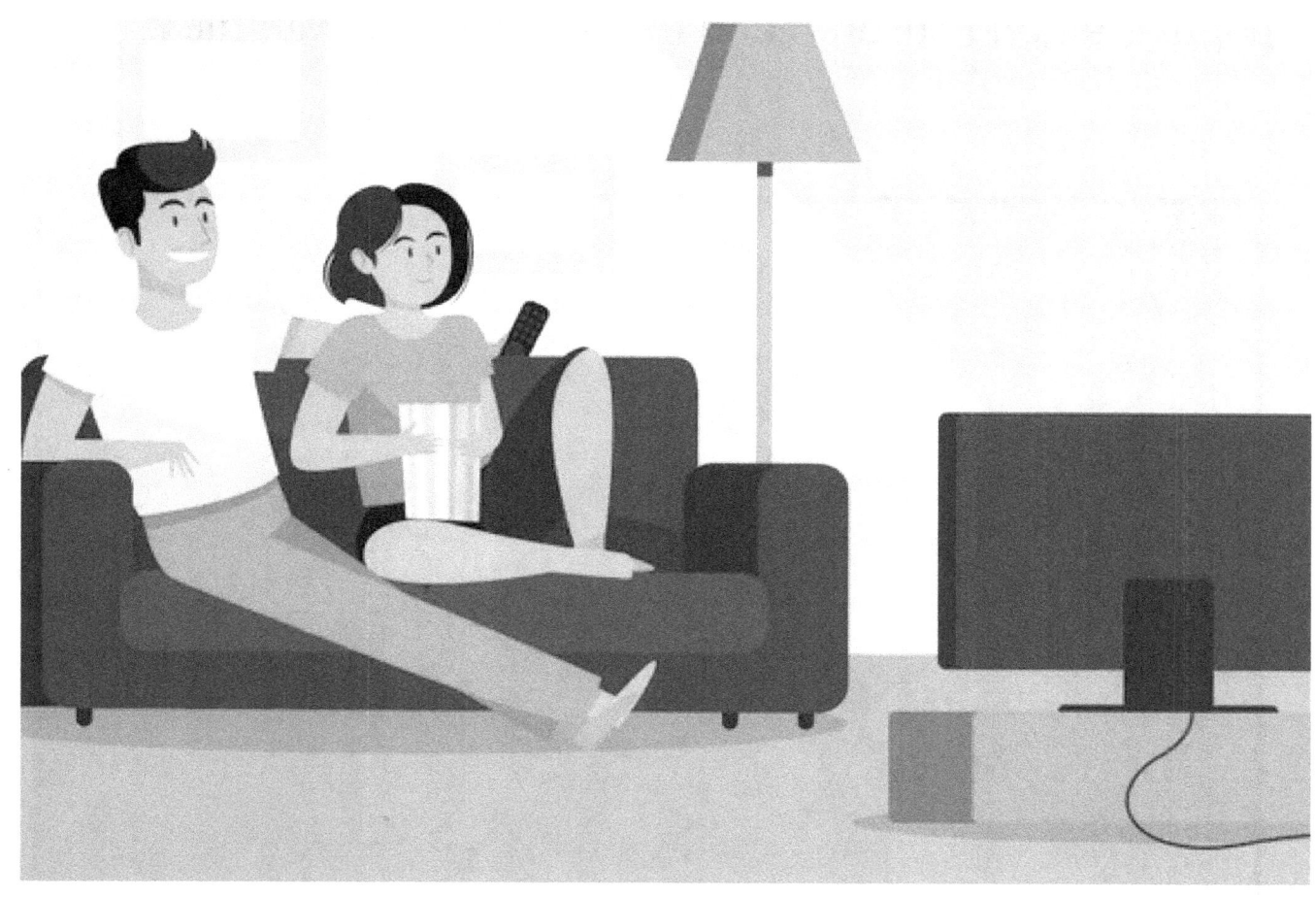

Sweetened Breakfast Cereals: Do not eat this super sweet treat. Breakfast cereals are processed cereal grains, such as wheat, oats, rice, and corn. They're especially popular among children and frequently eaten with milk.

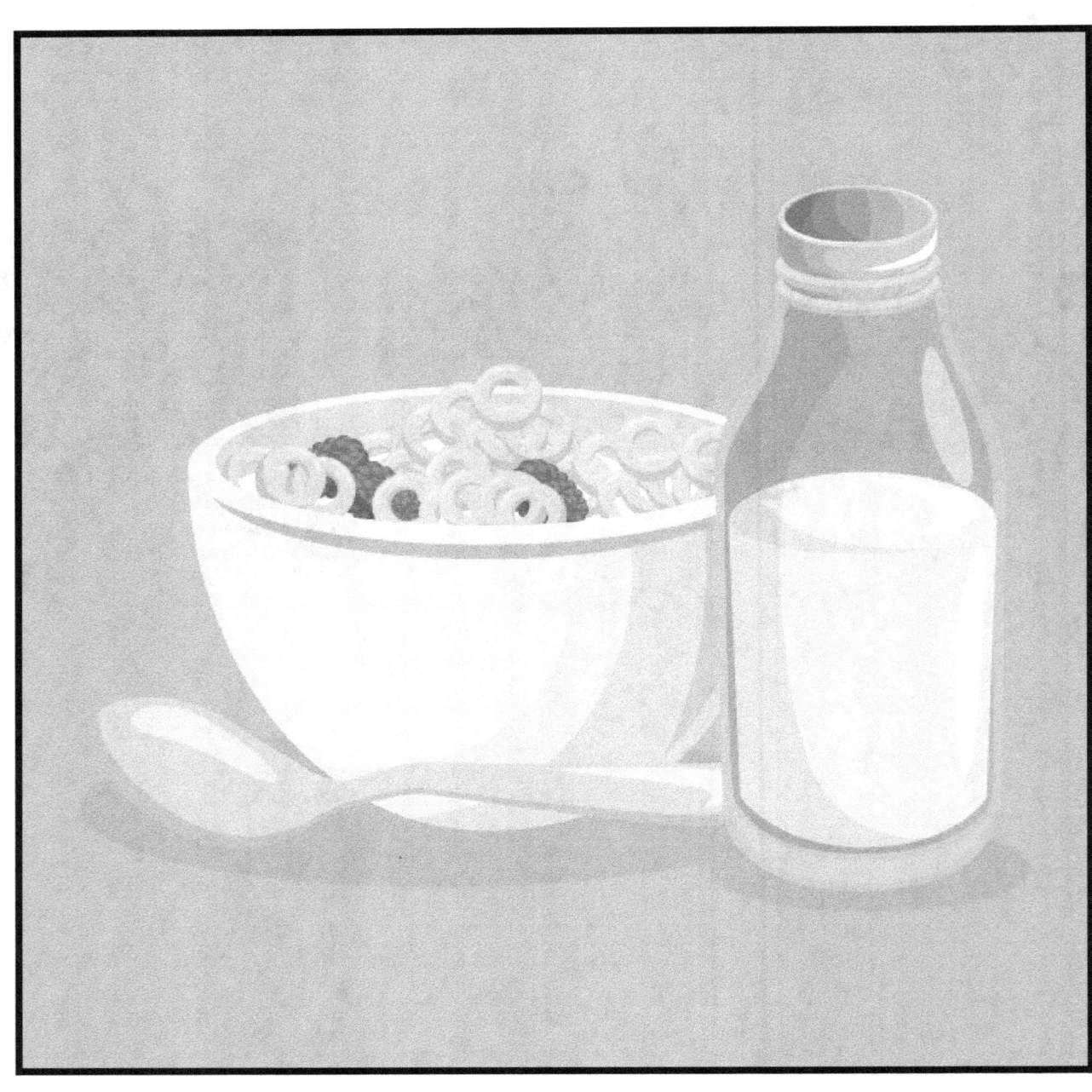

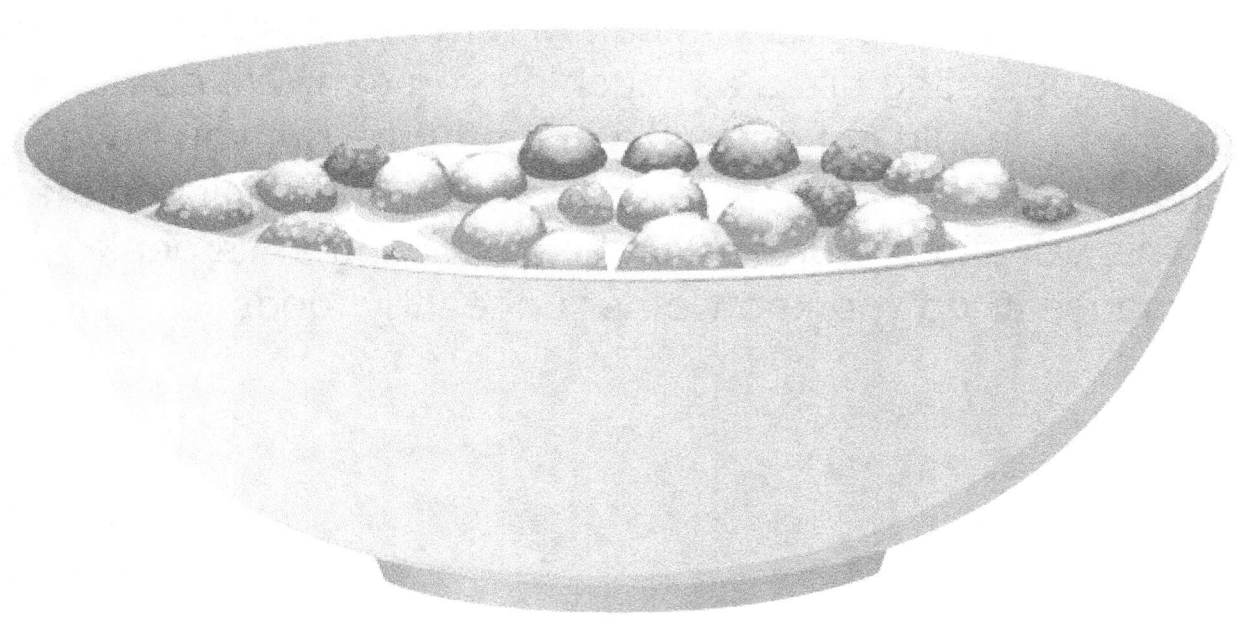

We've talked about what you can do to keep your body healthy by avoiding tons of foods that are not good for you at all. This will allow you to protect your health as much as you can in this day and age to remember that you need to avoid sugary drinks as much as you can to remember also that you have to avoid eating pizza as much as you can. We do not say that you should not eat pizza in the future but you have to consume less pizza then you have been consuming in the past. This will allow your body to keep working at its peak performance to do you know other unhealthy foods.

Disclaimer Statement

All information and content contained in this book are provided solely for general information and reference purposes. SSP LLC Limited makes no statement, representation, warranty or guarantee as to the accuracy, reliability or timeliness of the information and content contained in this Book.

Neither SSP Limited or the author of this book nor any of its related company accepts any responsibility or liability for any direct or indirect loss or damage (whether in tort, contract or otherwise) which may be suffered or occasioned by any person howsoever arising due to any inaccuracy, omission, misrepresentation or error in respect of any information and content provided by this book (including any third-party books.